Low FODMAP

A Beginner's Step-by-Step Guide To Reducing IBS Symptoms

With Recipes and a Meal Plan

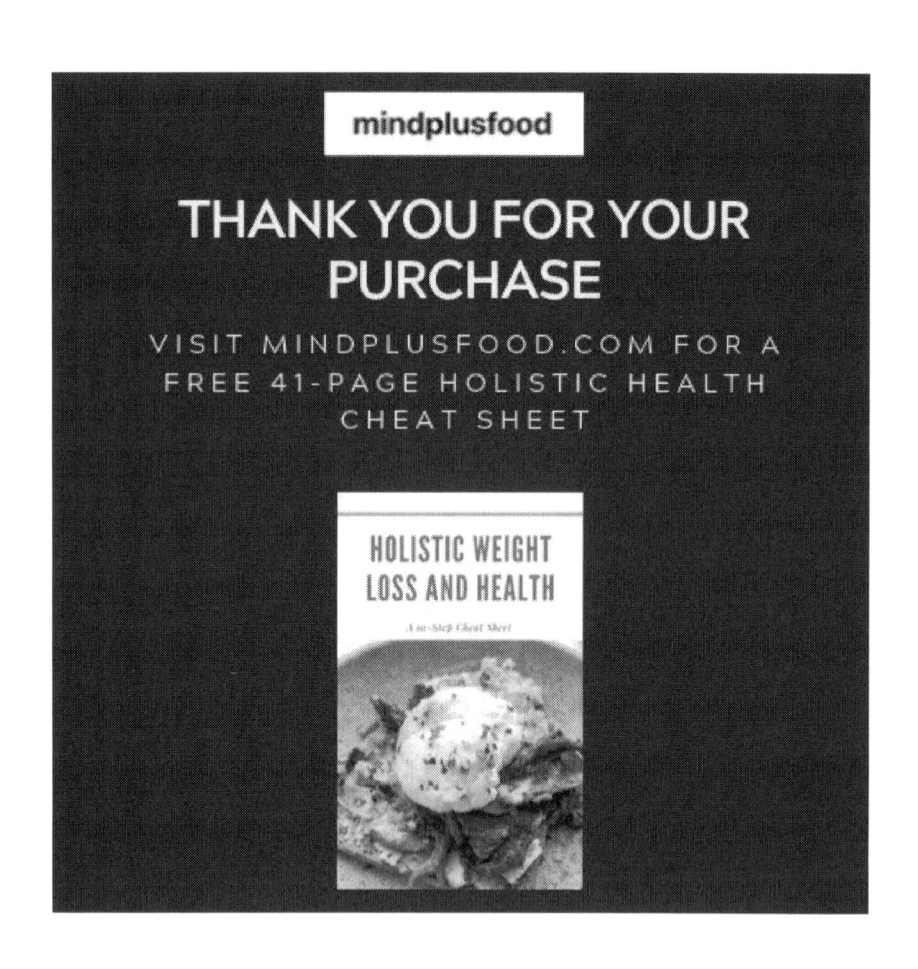

Copyright © 2019 Brandon Gilta

All rights reserved. No portion of this book may be reproduced in any form without permission from the publisher, except as permitted by U.S. copyright law.

Disclaimer

By reading this disclaimer, you are accepting the terms of the disclaimer in full. If you disagree with this disclaimer, please do not read the book. The content in this book is provided for informational and educational purposes only.

This book is not intended to be a substitute for the original work of this diet plan. At most, this book is intended to be beginner's supplement to the original work for this diet plan and never act as a direct substitute. This book, is an overview, review, and commentary of the facts of that diet plan.

All product names, diet plans, or names used in this book are for identification purposes only and are property of their respective owners. Use of these names does not imply endorsement. All other trademarks cited herein are property of their respective owners.

None of the information in this book should be accepted as independent medical or other professional advice.

The information in the books has been compiled from various sources that are deemed reliable. It has been analyzed and summarized to the best of the Author's ability, knowledge, and belief. However, the Author cannot guarantee the accuracy and thus should not be held liable for any errors.

You acknowledge and agree that the Author of this book will not be held liable for any damages, costs, expenses, resulting from the application of the information in this book, whether directly or indirectly. You acknowledge and agree that you assume all risk and responsibility for any action you undertake in response to the information in this book.

You acknowledge and agree that by continuing to read this book, you will (where applicable, appropriate, or necessary) consult a qualified medical professional on this information. The information in this book is not intended to be any sort of medical advice and should not be used in lieu of any medical advice by a licensed and qualified medical professional.

Always seek the advice of your physician or another qualified health provider with any issues or questions you might have regarding any sort of medical condition. Do not ever disregard any qualified professional medical advice or delay seeking that advice because of anything you have read in this book.

Table of Contents

Introduction 7

Chapter 1 – Small Intestinal Bacterial Overgrowth (SIBO) and Irritable Bowel Syndrome (IBS) 10

Chapter 2 – The Low FODMAP Diet 15

Chapter 4 – The Low-FODMAP Diet Program -Week 2 32

Chapter 5 - The Low-FODMAP Diet Program —Weeks 3 and 4 39

Conclusion 49

Introduction

I want to thank you and congratulate you for getting this guide.

This guide contains necessary information about the low-FODMAP diet that is becoming popular nowadays. This book also suggests an effective low-FODMAP diet program that will be beneficial to people with IBS and other digestive tract disorders.

SIBO, which stands for Small Intestinal Bacterial Overgrowth is a condition that results from too much bacterial growth in the gut. This condition causes abdominal pain, diarrhea, constipation, and abdominal distention to an affected person.

SIBO is believed to be one of the main causes of IBS or Irritable Bowel Syndrome. IBS is a gastrointestinal disease that has similar symptoms to SIBO.

IBS symptoms can cause anxiety and stress to a person which leads to overeating. Binge eating and stress eating can lead to high levels of FODMAPs -Fermentable Oligosaccharides, Disaccharides, Monosaccharides, And Polyols. FODMAPs are sugars or short-chain carbohydrates that are not easily absorbed in the small intestine. When they reach the large intestine, they accumulate gas and attract water that causes different symptoms. They can also produce toxic gases such as methane and hydrogen that cause different IBS symptoms.

This book also provides up-to-date information about the low-FODMAP diet and how it should be implemented. This also includes low-FODMAP recipes and a meal plan that you can use while on the diet program. Follow the suggested information present in this book to effectively manage your IBS symptoms. Most importantly, this book will teach you to take good care of your body by establishing an effective, beneficial, and healthy eating habits. When all else fails, consult your doctor.

Thanks again for getting this guide, I hope you enjoy it!

Chapter 1 – Small Intestinal Bacterial Overgrowth (SIBO) and Irritable Bowel Syndrome (IBS)

SIBO stands for Small Intestinal Bacterial Overgrowth. This is a condition that results from excessive bacterial growth in the small intestine. Normally, a healthy individual has a significantly low population of bacteria in the small intestine. When other bacteria that typically grow in other parts of the digestive tract start invading the small intestine, SIBO can happen. Small intestine bacterial overgrowth is more common in females, people 60 years old and above, and those with digestive tract disorders. Too much bacterial content in the small intestine can cause abdominal pain, diarrhea, and abdominal distention. Since the bacteria start sucking up the nutrients in the small bowel, this often leads to malnutrition.

Causes

The exact cause of small intestine bacterial overgrowth remains unknown. However, the following are believed to be the causes of this digestive tract disease:

- Anatomic abnormalities in the small intestine
- Acute or sudden changes in the small bowel
- pH changes in the small intestine
- A compromised or weakened immune system
- Low levels of hydrochloric acid or stomach acid
- Impaired muscular activity of the small intestine

Signs and Symptoms

Many SIBO symptoms are due to malabsorption of nutrients brought by bacterial overgrowth. These bacteria cause inflammation of the small bowel which impairs absorption and digestion processes.

The following are the signs and symptoms of Small Intestine Bacterial Overgrowth.

- Abdominal pain
- Queasiness
- Bloating
- Abdominal cramps
- Constipation
- Diarrhea
- Indigestion
- Nausea
- Flatus

- Increased permeability of the small intestine
- Weight loss
- Anemia

Risk Factors

The following are the things/conditions that can make a person at risk of SIBO:

- Age (50 years old and up)
- Previous surgery
- Drinking alcohol and smoking
- Celiac disease (gluten enteropathy)
- Diverticulosis
- Diabetes
- Crohn's disease
- Hypothyroidism
- HIV
- Scleroderma
- Fibromyalgia
- Medicines – narcotics, antibiotics, and Proton Pump Inhibitors (PPIs)

Diagnoses

People who have symptoms of SIBO may undergo the following diagnostic tests:

- ***D-Xylose Test***

Xylose is a kind of sugar that can be digested easily without the use of enzymes. D-Xylose test requires the patient to consume a certain amount of D-xylose sugar. After this, the doctor will measure the xylose levels in the patient's blood and urine. If there are traces of D-xylose in the urine and blood of the patient, he is more likely to have problems in his digestive tract.

- **Breath Tests**

Breath tests are used to measure the concentration of hydrogen, hydrogen sulfide, and methane in the patient's breath. These harmful gases are the products of carbohydrate breakdown in the gut. Different bacteria in the small intestine initiate and perform this breakdown. The poisonous gases can go to the bloodstream and will be carried by the blood vessels to different parts of the body – including the lungs. Before undergoing a breath test, the patient will be asked to do fasting for 24 hours. During the test, he will be given a glass of sugar lactulose. After consuming the drink, the patient will breathe into a balloon or a series of tubes for 2-3 hours at regular intervals. The results of breath tests will determine the location and severity of the bacterial overgrowth in the small intestine.

Treatments

Antibiotics are considered as the primary medical management for SIBO. Rifampicin is given to patients with high amounts of Hydrogen gas in their breath. Meanwhile, a combination of Rifampicin and Neomycin is given to patients with high levels of methane in their breath. It is necessary to ask the physician regarding the right kinds of antibiotics to be taken and their correct dosages. In some cases, surgery may be required especially when the intestinal structures are damaged.

SIBO and IBS

Irritable Bowel Syndrome (IBS) is a gastrointestinal (GI) disorder characterized by bloating and distention, abdominal pain, flatulence, diarrhea, and constipation. These symptoms can lead to unmanageable stress and anxiety that affect a person's normal life. Like SIBO, the exact cause of IBS remains unknown. But this gastrointestinal disorder is believed to be caused by the following:

- Inflammation in the intestine
- Impaired nerve functions in the digestive system

- Long and forceful contractions in the intestine
- Changes in the microflora or good bacteria in the gut
- Severe bacterial or viral infection in the intestine

According to different researches and studies, SIBO is **one of the possible causes of Irritable Bowel Syndrome or IBS**. But this remains a theory until today. It is assumed that 4% - 78% of patients diagnosed with IBS have small intestinal bacterial overgrowth (SIBO). At present, the medical community is still conducting various studies and researches to prove this claim.

Chapter 2 – The Low FODMAP Diet

FODMAPs are sugars or short-chain carbohydrates that are not easily absorbed in the small intestine. When they reach the large intestine, they accumulate gas and attract water that causes different symptoms.

These food carbs are being fermented by different kinds of bacteria in the gut. FODMAPs include fructose, lactose, sugar alcohols, short-chain oligosaccharide polymers. The majority of these carbs are naturally present in different foods and beverages we consume. Polyols are present in commercially-prepared food products and beverages in the market.

FODMAPs are considered as a dietary fiber because they are resistant to digestion. They will pass through the intestine without changing their natural components. When these sugar reaches the colon, they are fermented and utilized as fuel by the microflora or good intestinal bacteria.

FODMAPs can be beneficial to a person's overall health and well-being. However, the microflora tends to produce methane, a gas that can cause flatulence and bloating. Also, the bacteria that feed on these sugar (FODMAPs) can produce Hydrogen gas that can lead to abdominal pain, cramps, and constipation. These symptoms are mainly due to gut distention which makes your stomach appear big.

It is important to note that FODMAPs are not the real cause of Irritable Bowel Syndrome (IBS) and other similar conditions. However, limiting FODMAPs intake can help manage or reduce IBS and SIBO symptoms. These short-chain carbohydrates can cause digestive discomfort especially in people who are hypersensitive to luminal distension. But these carbs do not cause inflammation in the intestinal tract. It is medically proven that naturally occurring FODMAPs help prevent digestive discomfort.

Benefits of a Low FODMAP Diet

As the name implies, a low-FODMAP diet is a type of diet that limits the intake of foods that are high in FODMAPs. This diet was developed by a group of researchers at Monash University in Victoria. Low FODMAP diet helps people with IBS and SIBO manage their symptoms. This **research** shows that 75% of people with Irritable Bowel Syndrome can benefit from a low-FODMAP diet. The following are some of the many benefits of a low-FODMAP diet:

- Less gas and less bloating
- Improved bowel condition

- Reduced incidence of diarrhea and constipation
- Reduced stomach pain
- Increased quality of life

What to Eat

Bear in mind that a low-FODMAP diet aims not to eliminate FODMAPs. The goal of this diet is to reduce the intake of these short-chain carbohydrates to help manage the symptoms of digestive disorders. The following are the foods that you can safely eat on a low-FODMAP diet:

- ***All kinds of fats and oils***
- ***Eggs, meats, fish, tofu***
- ***Most herbs and spices*** – parsley, coriander, basil, thyme, tarragon, basil, cumin, turmeric, ginger, etc.
- ***Dairy Products*** – lactose-free dairy products (milk, yogurts, etc.), hard cheese, and aged softer varieties like camembert and brie
- ***Fruits*** – strawberries, blueberries, raspberries, bananas, cantaloupes, melons (except watermelon), grapes, lime, lemon, kiwi, mandarins, passionfruit
- ***Vegetables*** – bean sprouts, green beans, bok choy, alfalfa, cucumber, lettuce, choy sum, chives, carrots,

celery, eggplant, parsnips, potatoes, spinach, radishes, zucchini, squash, yams, turnips, tomatoes, green parts of the leek
- ✓ **Nuts and Seeds** – peanuts, cashews, almonds, pine nuts, macadamia nuts, sesame seeds
- ✓ **Bread and Cereals** – rice, potatoes, corn, maize, quinoa, flour-made bread (flour alone), spelt, oats, tapioca, sorghum
- ✓ **Beverages** – water, tea, coffee, etc.

What To Avoid

The following foods that are high in FODMAPs should be avoided or consumed in significantly low amounts:

- ❖ **Dairy Products** – regular milk (milk from cows, sheep, and goat), most yogurts, fresh cheeses (ricotta, cottage, etc.), ice cream, whey protein supplements
- ❖ **Legumes** – beans, lentils, baked beans, red kidney beans, soybeans, chickpeas
- ❖ **Fruits** – apples, cherries, apricots, peaches, pears, blackberries,

boysenberries, figs, dates, watermelon, canned fruits
- ❖ ***Vegetables*** – asparagus, shallots, artichokes, peas, broccoli, onions, beetroot, okra, Brussels sprouts, mushrooms, cabbage, leeks, fennel, cauliflower, cabbage
- ❖ ***Wheat*** – bread, biscuits, pasta, pancakes, waffles, breakfast cereals, tortillas
- ❖ ***Grains*** – rye, barley
- ❖ ***Sweeteners*** – honey, mannitol, sorbitol, maltitol, xylitol, fructose, high-fructose corn syrup
- ❖ ***Beverages*** – milk, soy milk, fruit juices, fortified wines, beer, soft drinks with high-fructose corn syrup

How to Follow a Low-FODMAP Diet

Before you undergo a low-FODMAP diet, you need to make a plan and develop a strategy. Ask your physician and dietician if you are eligible to take this kind of diet. Most importantly, you need to strictly follow the whole course of the diet program to achieve the desired results.

For best results, follow these tips:

- ✓ Strictly follow a low-FODMAP diet for 2-5 weeks. This means you will be

avoiding high-FODMAP foods for 14-35 days.
- ✓ After 2-5 weeks, you can reintroduce regular foods (high-FODMAPs) week by week. This will help you determine which type/s of foods cause/s the symptoms.
- ✓ Once you've found the real cause of your IBS or digestion disorder, completely avoid the food/s to prevent the symptoms from recurring.
- ✓ When all else fails, consult your doctor/dietician.

Considerations

Before taking the challenge, take note of the following:

1. ***IBS Diagnosis***

   There is no confirmatory test for irritable bowel syndrome. However, your doctor can diagnose your IBS based on specific criteria. It is extremely important to consult your doctor about your condition especially when you have signs of IBS and other digestive disorders. This is to rule out more serious gut diseases such as inflammatory bowel disease, celiac disease, and colon cancer. It is not recommended to take the low-FODMAP diet without the advice of a health professional.

   The doctor can confirm the IBS diagnosis based on these three official IBS diagnostic criteria:

   - Recurrent abdominal pain
   - Persistent symptoms
   - Changes in the appearance and frequency of the stool

2. ***First-Line Diet Strategies***

The low-FODMAP is considered as a second-line dietary program and is only ordered to people who refused to take the first-line strategies. To find out more about first-line dietary advice, visit this **site**.

3. ***Planning Strategies***

A SMART (Specific, Measurable, Attainable, Realistic, Timely) plan is needed to implement the diet program properly. List down all the things that you need to do in a piece of paper or a small notebook. Before buying all the ingredients, prepare a low-FODMAP shopping list. Study the low-FODMAP menus and recipes carefully to get the best results.

Chapter 3 – The Low-FODMAP Diet Program -Week 1

The low-FODMAP diet program is intended for people with irritable bowel syndrome and other digestive disorders such as SIBO. This kind of diet aims to know the kinds of low-FODMAP foods a person can tolerate and those that can trigger IBS symptoms. These things are necessary for developing a healthy, less-restrictive, and low-FODMAP meal plan that will help manage your condition.

The low-FODMAP diet is composed of three phases:

1. ***Phase 1 – Elimination***
   For 2-5 weeks of the diet program, you have to exclude all high-FODMAP foods from your diet. In this period, you will find alternative FODMAPs (low-FODMAP foods) that you will use throughout the diet program. For instance, if you are normally consuming milk and bread with cheese during breakfast, you can replace them with steamed potatoes and strawberries.
2. ***Phase 2 – Reintroduction***
   After the elimination period – which usually happens for 2-5 weeks, start

reintroducing high-FODMAP foods one at a time. You can do it weekly (one FODMAP per week) or every three days. In this phase, you will be able to find out the foods that cause IBS symptoms. Simply eliminate them from the diet and continue reintroducing.

3. ***Phase 3 – Adaptation***

   After identifying the cause of IBS symptoms, start formulating or developing a diet plan that will help manage your condition. Use the information to help manage your symptoms and live a better life. Just make sure your diet plan is approved by your physician and dietician.

The First Week

Week 1 is considered as the most critical week in the low-FODMAP diet program. This is the start of the elimination phase in which you will be eliminating FODMAPs from your diet. If you have allergies to certain food/s, inform your dietician and find alternatives. Expect for sudden changes in your bodily functions and consider them normal. These are part of the adaptation process. Do not give in to your cravings and strictly follow what's written in your diet plan. Then do the following:

1. ***Ask your physician and/or dietician.***
   Your IBS health care team knows all the things about your condition – history of disease, signs and symptoms, allergies, current medications, etc. They should be the very first people to know about your decision. If they think this kind of diet can harm your overall health and well-being, accept their decision. But if your team suggests that you need to undergo a low-FODMAP diet program, give it a go.
2. ***Make a weekly plan.***

A weekly plan will serve as your guide for the whole 7 days of taking the diet program. List all the menus and recipes that you are going to prepare for the whole week and study your plan. Also, list down all the necessary ingredients and cooking utensils/equipment to prevent unnecessary circumstances.

3. ***Choose water or some tea as drinks.***
   Remember that water is the safest drink to use in the diet program. Do not include carbonated drinks, fruit juices, and artificially-prepared juices in your diet. You can use black tea, green tea, and peppermint tea early in the morning or in the evening (before going to sleep). As much as possible, refrain from drinking any kind of milk.

4. ***Prepare a food diary.***
   A food diary will serve as your progress notes while on a low-FODMAP diet program. You can list down all the important things that happen in the diet program – common mistakes, important developments, foods that trigger IBS, etc.

Days 1, 2, 3

This guide highly suggests consuming the same sets of food recipes/menus for 3 days. This is to teach your body how to adapt to a sudden change in the usual food consumption process. This is also one of the best ways to learn how to love the new set of foods being introduced.

♦ *Breakfast*

Remember, breakfast is referred to as the most important meal of the day. You need to take a heavy breakfast meal to have sufficient energy throughout the day.

For days 1-3, eat the following foods during breakfast:
- Scrambled eggs
- 10 pcs (150 grams) medium-sized strawberries or 1 cup (150 grams)
  of grapes. *Note:* Grapes and strawberries contain 0 (zero) FODMAP.
- 1 medium-sized orange fruit (130 grams)
- 1 cup of black coffee
- 1 glass of freshwater

In making the perfect scrambled eggs, use this recipe as your guide:

"Scrambled Eggs"

Ingredients:

2 large eggs

6 tbsps. full cream milk (you can also use single cream milk)

a knob of unsalted butter

a pinch of salt

Instructions:

1. Whisk the 2 eggs in a bowl, then add the cream milk and salt. Mix thoroughly until the mixture becomes soft and smooth.
2. Heat a small non-stick pan over medium heat for 1-2 minutes. Add the butter and allow to melt.
3. Pour in the mixture and cook for 20 seconds without stirring. Using a wooden spoon, stir the mixture and fold it over from the bottom of the frying pan.
4. Allow to sit for 5-7 minutes and fold again. Stir again and serve hot.

⭐ Lunch

Forget about the meat first. Part of this low-FODMAP diet program is to eliminate all meat products (except eggs) for 3 days. This is because meat dishes can increase your appetite. Also, according to researches, some meat products can cause unmanageable stress that can lead to stress eating and binge eating.

For days 1 to 3, consume the following foods:
- Potato & Egg Salad
- 1/3 slice ripe banana, 20 pcs blueberries, ½ cup cantaloupe
- 1-2 glasses of water

"Potato and Egg Salad"

Ingredients:

800 g potato

4 large eggs

1 red bell pepper, diced

160 g green peas

1 small cucumber, cut into sticks

3 tbsps. fresh chives, chopped

3 tbsps. scallions/green onions (green tips only), chopped

1 tbsp. lemon juice

1 tbsp. wholegrain mustard

grind black pepper to season

1/3 cup mayonnaise

Instructions:

1. Wash the potatoes over running water and cut into bite-sized pieces. Cut the beans into small pieces and set aside.
2. Fill in a large saucepan with 5 cups of water and add the potatoes. Cook the potatoes over medium-high heat for 15-20 minutes or until soft and tender.
3. Add the green beans and cook for 3-5 minutes. Drain and set aside to cool.
4. Cook the eggs for 10-15 minutes or until hard, then cut into quarters.
5. In a small mixing bowl, mix thoroughly the mayonnaise, lemon juice, wholegrain mustard,

and black pepper. This will serve as your salad dressing.

6. Using a large mixing bowl, combine the potatoes, green peas, cucumber, green onions/scallions, red bell peppers, and chives. Add the salad dressing and season with grinds of black pepper. Mix well and serve.

Dinner

For the first three days of the low-FODMAP diet program, you can consume the following vegetable and fruit salads:

- **Greek Salad**
  Ingredients: 1 oz. feta cheese, romaine lettuce, 3-5 slices small cucumber, 5 black olives, ¼ cup cherry tomatoes.
  Simply combine all these ingredients in a large salad bowl and drizzle with 2 tbsps. extra-virgin olive oil. Season with salt and pepper and sprinkle with oregano. Then serve.

- ***Strawberry Blueberry Spinach Salad***
  In a large salad bowl, combine 5 chopped strawberries,

chopped blueberries, 1 ½ cups of baby spinach, 1 oz. crumbled goat cheese, and 4 crushed walnuts. In a separate bowl, prepare the salad dressing by mixing ½ tbsp. extra-virgin olive oil, cracked black pepper, and ½ tbsps. rice wine vinegar. Add the dressing to the large salad bowl and stir well, then serve.

Drink 1-2 glasses of water (not cold) after eating.

- **Snacks**
  - **40 g of mixed nuts – macadamias, walnuts, cashews, pine nuts, peanuts, etc.**
  - **1 glass of water**

After supper, do not eat anything – especially chips, chocolates, candies, and junk foods. Before sleeping, drink 1 cup of warm, unsweetened jasmine tea.

For the remaining days of the week, you can consume the following foods:

- **Breakfast**

    Aside from scrambled eggs and low-FODMAP berries, you can also eat low FODMAP blueberry pancakes, poached eggs on toast, and low FODMAP blueberry smoothie.

- Lunch

    You can now incorporate meat into your diet. You can also try cooking easy lunch recipes on this site.

- For dinner, we advise you to simply consume vegetable and fruit salads for good digestion and easy defecation. You can also try this easy salad recipe with meat:

    "Cobb Salad"

Ingredients:

   1 hardboiled egg
   3 oz. skinless, boneless chicken
   ¼ cup cherry tomatoes
   1 slice turkey bacon, crumbled
   feta cheese, crumbled

bibb lettuce
romaine lettuce
lemon juice
extra-virgin olive oil
herbs of your choice

Instruction:

Simply mix all the solid ingredients in a large salad bowl and add the salad dressing (a combination of olive oil, lemon juice, and herbs).

Chapter 4 – The Low-FODMAP Diet Program -Week 2

Week 2 is considered as the reinforcement week of the low-FODMAP diet. You need to introduce other menus and recipes to your usual meal plan (first-week menus) to get sufficient amounts of nutrients.

If the symptoms of IBS and other digestive tract disorders are relieved, it is an indication that the low-FODMAP diet works well in your body. It is important however to note that good eating habits alone cannot guarantee you the best results. Remember that stress is one of the major causes of IBS. You also need to practice relaxation activities to help manage IBS symptoms. A good exercise routine will also help you manage digestive tract disorders more effectively.

Recipes

Breakfast
- Breakfast recipes in week 1
- additional recipe: Lemon Loaf Cake
- black coffee or a glass of lactose-free milk

- a cup of lactose-free yogurt
- a glass of water

"Lemon Loaf Cake"

Ingredients:

For the loaf

1/3 c all-purpose flour plus more (for dusting)

1/3 c almond meal

2 tsp gluten-free baking powder

½ tsp xanthan gum

1 c olive oil

4 large eggs

2 tbsps. poppy seeds

½ c Great Lakes Gelatin Collagen Hydrolysate

½ cup of coconut sugar

½ tsp pure vanilla extract

1 lemon zest finely grated

¼ cup lemon juice

For the glaze

¼ c coconut butter

1 tbsp. lemon juice

2 tbsps. maple syrup

1 c water

½ tsp turmeric

½ tsp. vanilla

1/4 c Great Lakes Gelatin Collagen Hydrolysate

1 tsp lemon zest for garnish

Instructions:

1. Preheat the oven by setting the temperature to 350°F. Grease a 9x5-in loaf pan or line the pan with two pieces of parchment or wax paper.
2. Using a small mixing bowl, mix the flour, almond meal, xanthan gum, baking powder, and poppy seeds. Then set aside.
3. In a medium-sized mixing bowl, combine the olive oil, coconut sugar, maple syrup, and vanilla. Then add the eggs and mix well until smooth and soft in texture. Add the juice and lemon zest and

stir thoroughly until fully combined.
4. Add the flour mixture (small bowl) into the egg mixture and mix thoroughly. Then add the gelatin collagen hydrolysate and mix again for 10-15 minutes or until the mixture becomes soft and smooth.
5. Place the batter to the prepared pan and bake in the oven for 50-60 minutes or until the top is golden brown. Allow cooling.
6. Heat a small saucepan over low heat. Add the lemon juice, coconut butter, vanilla, maple syrup, water, turmeric, and Great Lakes Gelatin Collagen Hydrolysate. Stir the mixture carefully until smooth and silky.
7. Drizzle the cake with lemon glaze and cut into slices. Enjoy!

⊥ Lunch
- lunch recipes in week 1
- 1/3 slice ripe banana, 20 pcs blueberries, ½ cup cantaloupe, 1 medium-sized Mandarin, 2 small kiwis, ½ breadfruit

- additional recipe: Pork Loin Roast
- a glass of water

"Pork Loin Roast"

Ingredients:

2.5 kg pork loin roast

200 g risotto rice or medium-grain white rice

2 cups of chicken stock

1 ½ cups of leek (green tips only)

½ tsp dried thyme

1 tbsp. olive oil

1 cup of chopped fresh parsley

1 tbsp. garlic-infused oil

3 tbsps. pumpkin seeds

1 tsp dried oregano

rock salt (to season)

Instructions:

1. Heat the olive oil in a large saucepan over medium heat for

2-3 minutes. Sauté the leek tips and garlic for 3 minutes and add the white rice. Stir for 1-2 minutes.
2. Pour in the chicken stock and mix thoroughly or until the stock has absorbed into the white rice. Cook for 20-25 minutes or until sticky.
3. Remove the pan from the heat and add the parsley, scallions, thyme, oregano, and pumpkin seeds. Stir thoroughly and transfer to a bowl to cool.
4. Set the oven to 430°F fan bake function.
5. Rub the pork loin skin with extra-virgin olive oil and season with salt. Place the pork in a roasting tray and cook in the oven for 30 minutes.
6. Remove from the oven and baste with juices, then season again with some salt.
7. Set the oven to 390°F and roast again for 120-160 minutes. Cover the pork with tin foil to avoid burning.

8. Remove from the oven and serve with your favorite low-FODMAP veggies and cranberry sauce.

⁕ Dinner
- dinner recipes in week 1
- additional recipe: Salmon and Salsa Verde
- a glass of water

"Salmon and Salsa Verde"

Ingredients:

4 salmon fillets

1 x 25 g pack dill, roughly chopped

1 x 25 g roughly chopped pack chives

1 x 25 g roughly chopped pack flat-leaf parsley

1 x 25 g mint tough, stalks removed and roughly chopped

1 x 200 g tin green olives, drained and stuffed with anchovies

2 tbsps. caper

2 lemon juice

2 tbsps. toasted pine nut

1 ½ tbsps. wholegrain mustard

Optional: 1 red chopped red pepper, 175 g wild and basmati rice, 75 g toasted pine nut, 50g stoned marinated black Kalamata olive

Instructions:

1. Set the oven temperature to 200°C/fan 180°C/gas 6.
2. In a food processor, put the herbs, pine nuts, capers, lemon juice, and olives and pulse until roughly chopped. This is your salsa verde.
3. Place/arrange the salmon on a lightly oiled baking sheet. Squeeze over the remaining lemon juice and season with black pepper. Cook in the oven for 12-15 minutes or until fully cooked.
4. Pour in the salsa verde on top of the salmon fillets. Serve with brown rice.

✣ Snacks
- **40 g of mixed nuts – macadamias, walnuts, cashews, pine nuts, peanuts, etc.**
- **1 glass of water**

After supper, do not eat anything – especially chips, chocolates, candies, and junk foods. Before sleeping, drink 1 cup of warm, unsweetened jasmine tea, ginger tea, or chamomile tea.

Chapter 5 - The Low-FODMAP Diet Program –Weeks 3 and 4

In this low-FODMAP diet program, we consider weeks 3 and 4 as the reintroduction phase. In these weeks, you will be reintroducing high-FODMAP foods one at time. You will do it every 3 days. this will help you find out the foods that cause the IBS/SIBO symptoms. After finding out the cause of such symptoms, you will eliminate that particular FODMAP in your diet.

Meal Plan

You will be using the same breakfast, lunch, dinner recipes included in this low-FODMAP diet program. If you want to include other low-FODMAP recipes/menus endorsed by your dietician, feel free to do so. You can also add the following recipes:

"Baked Sea Bass and Lemon Dressing"

(Lunch/Dinner)

Ingredients:

4x100g/4oz sea bass fillets

3 tbsps. extra-virgin olive oil

2 tbsps. small capers

grated lemon zest (1 lemon)

2 tbsps. flat-leaf parsley, chopped

2 tsp. gluten-free Dijon mustard

Instructions:

1. Using a small mixing bowl, make a salad dressing by mixing the lemon juice, zest, mustard, capers, seasonings, and water. Do not include the parsley.

2. Preheat the oven by setting to 200°C/fan 200°C/gas 7.

3. Line the baking tray with parchment paper and place the fish fillets.

4. Brush the skin of the fish with some olive oil and sprinkle with salt.

5. Bake for 7-9 minutes or until the flesh flakes when tested with a fork or a knife.

6. Arrange the fish on a large serving plate and garnish with extra parsley leaves.

"Low FODMAP Burger"

Ingredients:

- 1.25 lbs. ground pork
- ¼ tsp allspice
- ½ tsp salt
- ½ tsp white pepper
- ½ tsp ground nutmeg
- ½ tsp caraway seeds
- ½ tsp ground ginger

Instructions:

1. Preheat the grill then prepare the patty.

2. Using a small mixing bowl, stir together the salt, pepper, allspice, nutmeg, and ginger until fully combined.

3. Place the ground in a large mixing bowl and add the spice mixture. Mix thoroughly until spices are evenly distributed to the pork. Make round, flat burger patties using the palm of your hands.

3. Grill the patties and serve with gluten-free buns and mustard sauce.

"Slow Cooker Dairy-Free Butter Chicken"

Ingredients:

2 lbs. boneless and skinless chicken breast, chopped into chunks

15 oz.-can full-fat coconut milk

15 oz.-can tomato sauce

2 tbsps. lemon juice

1 cinnamon stick

2 tbsps. coconut oil

1 tsp. sea salt

1 pc. chopped yellow onion

5 cloves minced garlic

1 tsp chili powder

½ tsp. cayenne powder

1 in-knob ginger, chopped

2 tsp. ground turmeric

1 tbsp. garam masala

1 tbsp. cumin

½ ground pepper

½ tsp. ground cinnamon

Directions:

1. Preheat a large skillet or saucepan over medium heat and add the oil. Sauté onion and garlic for 5 minutes, then add the turmeric, garam masala, ginger, salt, pepper, chili powder, cayenne, and cinnamon. Toss to combine all the spices. Cook for 1-2 minutes over low-medium heat.

2. Transfer the mixture into the slow cooker, then add the chicken and other spices – coconut milk, lemon juice, tomato sauce, and cinnamon. Cover and cook for 2-3 hours over high heat.

3. Serve hot and garnish with fresh cilantro and some lime juice.

Recipes with High-FODMAP Ingredients

To help you know the specific food/s that cause/s your IBS symptoms, you need to reintroduce high-FODMAP foods in your diet program. You can use the following recipes with some high-FODMAP ingredients:

1. "Steak with Mushroom Stroganoff"

Ingredients:

    4 oz. rib-eye steak

    3 tbsps. extra-virgin olive oil

    salt and pepper

    4 oz. whole mushrooms, quartered

1 large clove garlic, minced

1 tsp. fresh parsley, minced

3 tbsps. chicken stock, or as needed

1 ½ oz. hard cheese

¼ tsp. black pepper, for the sauce

¼ tsp Worcestershire sauce

Directions:

1. Using a skillet, heat half of the olive oil over medium-high heat. Sprinkle a pinch of salt and pepper over the steak then sear for 3-5 minutes. Set aside the steak. Using another pan, heat the rest of the olive oil and add the mushroom. Cook the mushroom until softened.

2. Adjust the heat to low then add the garlic. Cook again for 12-2 minutes. Add the chicken stock and stir.

3. Add the Worcestershire sauce, hard cheese, and pepper. Blend the mixture well until the cheese incorporates into the sauce.

4. Serve the steak then add the finished mushroom stroganoff mixture. Garnish with parsley for presentation.

In this particular recipe, the <u>mushroom</u> is considered as a high-FODMAP food.

2. Creamy Low-FODMAP Fish Casserole"

Ingredients:

    1 ½ lb white fish, serving-sized pieces

    2 tbsps. olive oil

    2 tbsps. small capers

    1 lb. broccoli

    1 oz. grass-fed butter (for greasing)

    6 scallions

    1 lb. broccoli

    2 tbsps. small capers

    3 oz. grass-fed butter

    1 tbsp. Dijon mustard

    1 tbsp. dried barley

    1 tsp salt

    ¼ tsp ground black pepper

Directions:

1. Set the oven temperature to 400°F.

2. Cut the broccoli into small florets with the stems included. Fry the broccoli for 3-5 minutes until soft and golden, then add salt and pepper.

3. Add the finely chopped scallions and the capers, then fry for another 2-3 minutes.

4. Grease the baking dish with butter and add in the fried vegetables.

5. Add the white fish to the vegetable mix.

6. In an oven-ready plate, mix the parsley, mustard, and whipping cream. Add the fish and vegetable mix and top with some butter.

7. Bake for 20-30 minutes or until fully-cooked then serve.

In this particular recipe, <u>broccoli</u> is considered a high-FODMAP vegetable.

3. "Ground Beef Stroganoff"

Ingredients:

      1 lb. 80% lean ground beef

2 tbsp. butter

1 clove garlic, minced

10 oz. sliced mushrooms

1 tbsp. fresh parsley, chopped

1 tbsp. fresh lemon juice

salt and pepper to taste

2 tbsps. water

Directions:

1. Heat the large skillet over medium heat. Put the butter and let it melt, then add the garlic. When the garlic turns brown, add the beef and season with salt and pepper.

2. Drain some of the oil from the skillet and leave some to cook the mushroom.

3. Add the mushroom and cook for 2 minutes, then add the water. When the water is reduced to half, add the sour cream and paprika.

4. Reduce the heat temperature to low and add the lemon juice.

5. Garnish with parsley and serve immediately.

In this particular recipe, <u>mushroom and butter</u> are considered high-FODMAP foods.

You can also use other recipes containing high-FODMAP foods if you want to know the cause of your IBS.

After identifying the FODMAPs that cause your IBS symptoms, the next thing to do is to devise a meal plan that will help you manage your IBS symptoms more effectively.

This meal plan should include tolerable amounts of high-FODMAP foods to bring back flavors in your foods. The goal of the low-FODMAP diet program is not to eliminate high-FODMAP foods in the diet. Only those that trigger and worsen your IBS symptoms should be eliminated. After all, these so-called high FODMAPs are actually the most flavorful kinds of food in the world.

Conclusion

The Low FODMAP diet is a type of diet that is used to manage IBS symptoms. Limiting high-FODMAP intake can help manage or reduce IBS and SIBO symptoms. These short-chain carbohydrates can cause digestive discomfort especially in people who are hypersensitive to luminal distension. It is essential to know the specific FODMAPs that trigger your IBS symptoms to prevent the symptoms from recurring.

The low-FODMAP diet program is developed to help people with IBS and other digestive disorders manage their condition. This diet program can provide a person alternative IBS treatment that does not require too much medical attention. If you are suffering from SIBO/IBS conditions, do not hesitate to seek alternative treatments like a low-FODMAP diet. Most importantly, follow the advice of your physician and dietician. They know better about your condition.

Thank you again for getting this guide!

If you found this guide helpful, please take the time to share your thoughts and post a review. It'd be greatly appreciated!

Thank you and good luck!

mindplusfood

THANK YOU FOR YOUR PURCHASE

VISIT MINDPLUSFOOD.COM FOR A FREE 41-PAGE HOLISTIC HEALTH CHEAT SHEET

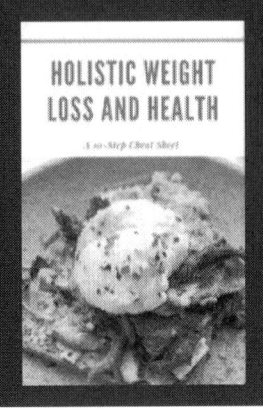

Printed in Great Britain
by Amazon